The definitive guide to PCOS (Polycystic Ovary Syndrome)

The Complete beginners guide with PCOS Managing Happiness and Health

Evelyn Pascal

1

PCOS Managing Happiness and Health

The purpose of this book

The purpose of this book is to empower individual with PCOS to manage their health and wellbeing.

PCOS definition (Polycystic Ovary Syndrome)

The appearance of many ovarian cysts, irregular menstruation periods, and elevated levels of androgens (male hormones) in the body are the hallmarks of PCOS, a common hormonal condition. It is a complicated illness that impacts women who are fertile in terms of their hormone, metabolic, and reproductive systems. PCOS frequently manifests as a variety of symptoms, such as weight gain, acne, hirsutism excessive development of facial and body hair and irregular or nonexistent periods. Long-term health problems include infertility, insulin resistance, type 2 diabetes, cardiovascular disease, and mood disorders are also linked to PCOS. Although the precise etiology of PCOS is unknown, genetics, insulin resistance, and hormone abnormalities are known to contribute to its development. A combination of the patient's medical history, physical examination, hormone level-assessing blood tests, and ultrasound imaging to determine ovarian morphology are usually used in the diagnosis process. Treatment strategies for PCOS include lifestyle changes, medicine, and occasionally assisted reproductive technology with the goals of controlling symptoms, regulating menstrual cycles, improving fertility outcomes, and lowering long-term health concerns.

Prevalence and effects on women's health

One of the most prevalent hormonal conditions affecting women who are fertile, PCOS (polycystic ovarian syndrome) has a serious negative influence on their health and general well-being. Depending on the diagnostic standards and population under study, PCOS's prevalence varies, but globally, it is thought to impact 5% to 20% of women.

The illness may significantly affect a number of facets of women's health, including:

1. Reproductive Health: Because of irregular or nonexistent ovulation, PCOS is a major factor in female infertility. In order to become pregnant, women with PCOS may find it difficult to conceive naturally and may need to use assisted reproductive technologies such in vitro fertilization (IVF) or ovulation induction.

2. Menstrual irregularities: One of the main indicators of PCOS is irregular menstrual cycles, which can include irregular timing of periods, protracted cycles, or even amenorrhea (lack of menstruation). These abnormalities can cause emotional discomfort and make family planning difficult.

3. Hyperandrogenism: Excessive facial and body hair, acne, and male-pattern baldness are signs of PCOS caused by elevated amounts of androgens, or male hormones. The quality of life and self-esteem may be affected by these outward expressions.

4. Metabolic Health: Insulin resistance, obesity, dyslipidemia, and a higher risk of type 2 diabetes are among the metabolic abnormalities that are intimately linked to PCOS. Specifically, insulin resistance has a role in weight gain and makes it harder to maintain a healthy weight.

5. Cardiovascular Health: Compared to

women without PCOS, women with the disorder are more likely to experience cardiovascular disease (CVD). Chronic inflammation, obesity, insulin resistance, dyslipidemia, hypertension, and hypertension are among the conditions linked to this higher risk.

6. Psychological Well-Being: An increased risk of mental disorders such as anxiety, depression, and low self-esteem is linked to PCOS. Psychological discomfort can be exacerbated by physical symptoms, fertility issues, and long-term health concerns.

Chapter two

Signs and standards for diagnosis of PCOS

Polycystic Ovary Syndrome, or PCOS, is a multifaceted hormonal condition with a wide range of indications and symptoms. Clinical presentation, medical history, physical examination, and laboratory testing are commonly used in the diagnosis of PCOS. An outline of the signs and diagnostic standards is provided below:

1. Menstrual irregularities are a common sign of polycystic ovary syndrome (PCOS). Period irregularities, protracted menstrual cycles, or amenorrhea (lack of menstruation) are possible manifestations of this. Menstrual abnormalities are commonly the result of inconsistent or missing ovulation in women with PCOS.

2. Hyperandrogenism: Women with PCOS, who have elevated amounts of androgens, or male hormones, may experience a range of symptoms, including:

• **Hirsutism:** Excessive development of facial and body hair, usually in the upper lip, chin, chest, and back areas, according to a male pattern.

• **Acne:** Enhanced cases of acne vulgaris, especially on the cheeks, forehead, and upper back.

• **Male-pattern Baldness:** Hair thinning on the scalp that resembles androgenic alopecia, also known as male-pattern baldness.

3. Polycystic Ovaries: Contrary to what the name implies, not all PCOS-affected women experience numerous ovarian cyst developments. However, polycystic ovaries can appear larger and contain many tiny follicles, giving them a distinctive appearance when examined with an ultrasound.

4. Other Indications and Symptoms:

• **Weight Gain:** Gaining weight is common in PCOS-affected women, particularly in the midsection.

• **Insulin Resistance:** Often associated with PCOS, insulin resistance can cause acanthosis nigricans, a darkening and thickening of the skin, particularly in body folds, and may also increase the risk of type 2 diabetes.

• **Mood Disorders:** An increased risk of mood disorders like anxiety and depression is linked to PCOS.

Diagnostic Criteria: The Rotterdam criteria, which demand the presence of at least two of the following three criteria, are one set of guidelines that are commonly used to diagnose PCOS.

1. Menstrual irregularities include irregular cycles, which can result in amenorrhea, or no menstruation at all, or oligomenorrhea, or infrequent menstruation because of insufficient ovulation.

2. Hyperandrogenism: Indications of increased androgen levels in the body, such as biochemical markers for hirsutism, acne, or male-pattern baldness.

3. Polycystic Ovaries: Polycystic ovaries are identified by ultrasound examination as having a volume larger than 10 mL and having 12 or more follicles in each ovary, each measuring 2 to 9 mm in diameter. Prior to confirming the diagnosis of PCOS, other possible reasons of hyperandrogenism and irregular menstruation should be considered. To accurately diagnose and treat PCOS, a complete medical history, physical examination, and the right laboratory testing are necessary.

Chapter three

Causes and Contributing elements

Although the precise origins of PCOS, or polycystic ovary syndrome, are unknown, a mix of environmental, hormonal, and genetic variables are thought to be involved. There are a number of known contributory elements that may interact differently in various people. The following are some of the main variables linked to the emergence of PCOS:

1. Genetic Predisposition: Research indicates that a substantial portion of PCOS development is likely influenced by heredity. PCOS is more common in women who have a family history of the disorder. Numerous genes, including those related to ovarian function, insulin signaling, and hormone regulation, have been linked to PCOS.

2. Hormonal imbalance: The hallmark of PCOS is an excess of androgens (male hormones) such as testosterone, as well as abnormalities in the synthesis and control of other hormones like insulin, follicle-stimulating hormone (FSH), and luteinizing hormone (LH). These hormone imbalances have the potential to impair ovarian function, which can result in ovarian cyst development, anovulation (absence of ovulation), and irregular menstrual periods.

3. Insulin Resistance: A typical characteristic of PCOS is insulin resistance, which results in compensatory hyperinsulinemia (higher insulin levels) as a result of the body's cells being less sensitive to the effects of insulin. A number of PCOS symptoms, such as hyperandrogenism, ovarian dysfunction, and metabolic disorders like obesity and dyslipidemia, can be attributed to insulin resistance. Hormonal imbalances can also be made worse by elevated insulin levels, which can cause the ovaries to produce more androgens.

4. Inflammation: The pathophysiology of PCOS has been linked to persistent low-grade inflammation. Women with PCOS have been shown to have elevated levels of pro-inflammatory cytokines and inflammatory markers such C-reactive protein (CRP). Insulin resistance, ovarian dysfunction, and other metabolic disorders linked to PCOS may be exacerbated by inflammation.

5. Environmental variables: A person's food, way of life, exposure to substances that disrupt hormones, stress, and other environmental variables can all have an impact on the onset and course of PCOS. Chronic stress, sedentary lifestyles, and high-calorie diets can all worsen insulin resistance and metabolic dysfunction. Exposure to specific environmental contaminants can also impair ovarian function and hormonal balance.

6. Gut Microbiota: New research indicates that dysbiosis, or changes in the gut microbiota, may be a factor in the onset of PCOS. Women with PCOS have been shown to have altered gut microbiota composition and function, which may be related to the inflammation and metabolic problems that are linked to the illness.

Early detection and detection are crucial.

For the reasons listed below, it is imperative that PCOS (Polycystic Ovary Syndrome) be identified and diagnosed as soon as possible:

1. **Preventing Long-Term Health Complications:** Endometrial cancer, type 2 diabetes, PCOS, and infertility are just a few of the long-term health issues that are linked to the syndrome. The implementation of suitable therapies to control symptoms, reduce health risks, and stop or postpone the onset of these consequences is made possible by early detection.

2. Improved Fertility Outcomes: Because of irregular menstrual cycles and ovulation, infertility is a significant worry for people with PCOS. Timely therapies to restore ovulation and enhance reproductive outcomes are made possible by early diagnosis. Many PCOS women can become pregnant successfully with the right care.

3. Handling Symptoms: Polycystic Ovary Syndrome (PCOS) can result in a number of symptoms that impair quality of life, such as irregular menstrual periods, hirsutism (overgrowth of hair), acne, weight gain, and mood swings. Early diagnosis enables the start of focused therapy to successfully manage these symptoms, enhancing general health and quality of life.

4. Preventing Metabolic Complications: Common metabolic abnormalities linked with PCOS include insulin resistance, obesity, dyslipidemia, and metabolic syndrome. Through medicine, targeted therapies, and lifestyle changes, early detection and management can help prevent or delay the advancement of many metabolic problems.

5. Personalized Treatment Planning: Because PCOS is a diverse disorder, there can be significant individual variation in the presentation and severity of symptoms. Early diagnosis improves treatment outcomes and adherence by enabling healthcare professionals to create individualized treatment programs that are catered to the unique requirements and objectives of each patient.

6. Taking Care of the Psychological Effects: Having PCOS can have a major psychological effect, which increases the risk of anxiety, depression, and low self-esteem. Healthcare professionals can address psychological and emotional needs, offer support, and connect patients with appropriate services like counseling or support groups when symptoms are detected and   diagnosed   early.

7. Patients are empowered when they are informed, and a timely diagnosis of PCOS helps them comprehend the disease, its effects, and their options for treatment. Patients who feel empowered are more likely to take an active role in their care, make wise decisions, and embrace healthy lifestyle choices that will improve their long-term health.

Nutrition and Diet

In order to effectively treat PCOS (Polycystic Ovary Syndrome), diet and nutrition are essential since they have a direct impact on hormone balance, insulin sensitivity, weight control, and general wellbeing. Here are some important things to think about when it comes to nutrition and food in PCOS patients:

1. Balanced macronutrients diet, such as having enough protein, good fats, and complex carbohydrates. Even distribution of macronutrients throughout the day can assist in lowering insulin resistance and stabilizing blood sugar levels.

2. Low Glycemic Index (GI) Foods: To reduce blood sugar spikes, select carbohydrates with a low GI. Whole grains, legumes, non-starchy vegetables, and fruits like citrus, berries, and apples are examples of low-GI foods.

3. Consume a wide variety of foods high in fiber, such as fruits, vegetables, whole grains, legumes, and nuts, as part of your diet. Fiber supports digestive health, encourages satiety, lowers blood sugar, and may help with weight management.

4. Healthy Fats: Consume foods high in avocados, nuts, seeds, olive oil, and fatty seafood like sardines and salmon as well as other sources of healthy fats. Essential fatty acids are provided by healthy fats, which also assist in hormone production and satiety maintenance.

5. Lean Protein: Choose protein sources that are low in fat, like fish, chicken, tofu, tempeh, lentils, and low-fat dairy. Protein supports the health of muscles, lowers blood sugar levels, and increases feelings of fullness.

6. Reduce Your Intake of Processed Foods and Added Sugars: Cut back on your intake of refined and processed foods, sweet snacks, desserts, sugary drinks, and meals with added sugars. Hormonal abnormalities, weight gain, and insulin resistance can all be attributed to these foods.

7. Portion Control: Be mindful of serving sizes to prevent overindulging. Smaller, more frequent meals spread out throughout the day can help control blood sugar levels and limit overindulgence in calories.

8. Timing of Meals: Try to eat at regular intervals and refrain from missing meals, particularly breakfast. Having breakfast within an hour of waking up can help control hunger hormones and accelerate metabolism.

9. Hydration: Throughout the day, make sure you drink lots of water to stay hydrated. Reduce your intake of sugary drinks and replace them with water, herbal teas, or infused water.

10. Customized Approach: Dietary requirements can differ amongst individuals with PCOS due to its diverse nature. In order to create a customized nutrition plan that meets your unique needs, tastes, and objectives, think about collaborating with a registered dietitian or other healthcare professional.

11. Supplementation: Taking supplements containing certain nutrients, like chromium, omega-3 fatty acids, inositol, and vitamin D, may help control the symptoms of PCOS in certain situations. see your doctor before beginning any supplement regimen.

12. Lifestyle Factors: Maintaining a healthy weight, managing stress, getting enough sleep, and engaging in regular physical activity are all crucial aspects of managing PCOS in addition to food. Combining these food adjustments with lifestyle adjustments might enhance general health and wellbeing even more.

Chapter four

Understanding the function of insulin resistance

In the context of PCOS (Polycystic Ovary Syndrome), an understanding of the role of insulin resistance is essential, as it is a fundamental aspect of the disorder and contributes too many of its symptoms and problems. An outline of insulin resistance and PCOS relevance is provided below:

1.The pancreas secretes the hormone insulin, which is essential for controlling blood sugar levels and promoting the uptake of glucose by cells for energy synthesis. Your body releases insulin in response to carbohydrate consumption, which aids in the movement of circulatory glucose into cells where it can be stored for later use or used as fuel.

2. Insulin Resistance Definition: Insulin resistance is the result of the body's cells losing their sensitivity to the actions of insulin, which impairs the absorption of glucose and raises blood sugar levels. The pancreas generates more insulin in response to this resistance, which raises blood levels of insulin above normal.

3. Insulin resistance is closely associated with PCOS: up to 70–80% of women with PCOS have insulin resistance. It is thought to be a major underlying cause of numerous metabolic and reproductive disorders linked to PCOS, such as:

- **Hyperandrogenism:** Excess androgens (male hormones) produced by the ovaries as a result of insulin resistance can cause symptoms like male-pattern baldness, hirsutism, and excessive hair growth.
- **Ovulatory Dysfunction:** Insulin resistance can cause irregular menstrual periods, anovulation (absence of ovulation), and infertility by interfering with the natural process of ovulation.

- **Metabolic Abnormalities:** Obesity, dyslipidemia (abnormal lipid levels), and a higher risk of type 2 diabetes and cardiovascular disease are all intimately associated with insulin resistance.

- Inflammation: Chronic low-grade inflammation linked to insulin resistance may worsen metabolic and reproductive abnormalities in PCOS.

4. Insulin resistance and hyperinsulinemia, or high insulin levels, can worsen hormonal imbalances and metabolic disorders associated with polycystic ovary syndrome (PCOS), leading to a vicious cycle of hyperandrogenism, insulin resistance, and metabolic dysfunction.

5. Impact on Treatment: One of the most crucial aspects of treating PCOS is managing insulin resistance. Dietary, physical activity and weight control adjustments are examples of lifestyle changes that can lower insulin levels and increase insulin sensitivity.

Moreover, drugs like insulin-sensitizing medicines (like metformin) may be administered to treat insulin resistance and enhance PCOS patients' metabolic and reproductive outcomes.

Importance of regular exercise in managing PCOS

For those with PCOS (Polycystic Ovary Syndrome), regular exercise has many advantages that can help with many elements of the disorder as well as general health and well-being. The following are some of the main advantages of consistent exercise for PCOS management:

1. Enhances Insulin Sensitivity: Exercise helps enhance insulin sensitivity, which makes it possible for cells to react to insulin more effectively and absorb glucose from the bloodstream more efficiently. This can lessen blood sugar levels, lessen insulin resistance, and minimize the chance of type 2 diabetes in PCOS patients.

2. Helps with Weight Management: Exercise is a useful tactic for encouraging weight loss and maintenance in PCOS patients, particularly those who are obese or overweight. Frequent exercise improves body composition and weight management by boosting metabolic rate, burning calories, and building lean muscle mass.

3. Controls Menstrual Cycles: For women with PCOS, exercise can help control their menstrual cycles and encourage ovulation. Frequent exercise can help balance hormones, lower excess androgens (male hormones), and enhance reproductive health, which can result in more regular menstrual cycles and higher fertility.

4. Lowers Androgen Levels: It has been demonstrated that exercise lowers the levels of androgens, or male hormones, in the blood in women with PCOS, which may help ease symptoms including acne, male-pattern baldness, and hirsutism, or excessive hair growth. Reproductive success and ovulatory function may both be enhanced by reducing androgen levels.

5. Reduces Cardiovascular Risk: Because of conditions like insulin resistance, obesity, dyslipidemia, and hypertension, PCOS is linked to a higher risk of cardiovascular disease (CVD). Frequent exercise reduces the risk of cardiovascular disease (CVD) in people with PCOS by lowering blood pressure, lowering cholesterol, increasing blood vessel function, and enhancing heart health.

6. Enhances Mood and Mental Health: Exercise has a positive impact on mood and can help reduce the tension, anxiety, and depressive symptoms that PCOS sufferers frequently face. Engaging in physical activity triggers the brain's release of feel-good neurotransmitters, such as endorphins, which enhance psychological comfort and well-being.

7. Boosts Energy: People with PCOS who regularly exercise can feel less tired and have more energy. Physical activity helps increase general health, endurance, and stamina, which improves quality of life and makes daily tasks easier to complete.

8. Promotes Bone Health: Women with PCOS may be more susceptible to bone loss because of hormonal imbalances and metabolic abnormalities linked to the disorder. Weight-bearing and resistance training can help strengthen bones and lower the risk of osteoporosis in these women.

9. Improves Quality of Life: For those with PCOS, exercise is beneficial to general health, vitality, and quality of life. Regular physical activity can have a good impact on many aspects of everyday life and give people the tools they need to better manage their illness by increasing physical fitness, lowering symptoms, and boosting psychological well-being.

Chapter five

Exercises that are appropriate for people with PCOS

Exercises that improve cardiovascular health, strength, flexibility, and general well-being are beneficial for those with PCOS (Polycystic Ovary Syndrome). It's critical to select exercises that are sustainable, pleasurable, and suitable for each person's fitness level and tastes. The following workout regimens are appropriate for people with PCOS:

1.Exercises for the Heart:

• **Brisk Walking:** Easily incorporated into daily life, walking is a low-impact aerobic workout. To strengthen your heart and burn calories, try to walk for at least 30 minutes most days of the week at a brisk pace.

• **Cycling:** Cycling is a fantastic cardiovascular exercise that is easy on the joints, whether it is done outside or on a stationary cycle. For a fun and practical approach to increase your fitness, consider adding cycling to your regimen.

• **Swimming:** This whole-body, low-impact activity improves cardiovascular health without straining joints. Engaging in water aerobics programs or swimming laps can enhance muscle tone and endurance.

• **Dancing:** Dancing is a lighthearted and entertaining approach to increase heart rate and burn calories. Dancing, whether it is hip-hop, salsa, or Zumba, has positive effects on the heart and emotions.

2. Strengthening Exercise:

• **Bodyweight Exercises:** You can perform exercises like planks, squats, lunges, and push-ups with just your body weight and with very little equipment. Exercises with only your bodyweight can boost your metabolism, increase muscular tone, and build strength.

• **Resistance Band Workouts:** You may target different muscle areas using resistance bands, which are a handy and adaptable workout tool. Exercises using resistance bands can help you define your muscles and gain strength.

• **Weightlifting:** Using weight machines or lifting weights at the gym can help increase metabolic rate, develop lean muscle mass, and enhance general strength and endurance. As you advance, progressively increase the intensity of the weights you start with.

3. Exercises for Flexibility and Balance:

• **Yoga:** Yoga enhances flexibility, balance, and relaxation by combining strength, flexibility, and mindfulness. Regular yoga practice helps ease tension in the muscles, enhance posture, and lower stress levels.

• **Pilates:** Using deliberate movements and breath work, Pilates focuses on developing core strength, stability, and flexibility. Pilates exercises can aid with core strengthening, posture correction, and general body awareness improvement.

- **Tai Chi:** Tai Chi is a gentle martial art that focuses on deep breathing and slow, flowing movements. Because it enhances balance, coordination, and relaxation, tai chi is appropriate for people of all fitness levels.

4. HIIT, or high-intensity interval training

- High-intensity interval training (HIIT) alternates short bursts of high-intensity exercise with rest or low-intensity activity. Exercises including high-intensity interval training (HIIT) are a great way to increase metabolism, improve cardiovascular fitness, and burn calories. HIIT should be used cautiously by PCOS sufferers, particularly if they have underlying medical issues or are inexperienced with exercise. As your fitness level rises, start with shorter intervals and progressively increase the length and intensity.

5. Body-Mind Techniques:

• **Mindfulness and meditation:** Mind-body techniques that assist lower stress, elevate mood, and enhance general wellbeing include mindfulness, deep breathing exercises, and meditation. Include these techniques in your daily routine to improve emotional equilibrium and relaxation.

• **Breathing Techniques:** Deep breathing techniques, such diaphragmatic or belly breathing can assist in triggering the body's relaxation reaction and lowering stress-related hormones. To encourage relaxation and reduce tension, consistently engage in deep breathing exercises.

It's crucial to pay attention to your body's signals and select pleasurable and comfortable **workouts.** Before beginning any new fitness program, speak with a healthcare professional. This is especially important if you haven't been active in a while or if you have any underlying health concerns. Start out softly and increase intensity and duration gradually. In addition, think about collaborating with a personal trainer or licensed fitness professional to create a safe and efficient workout program customized to your unique requirements and objectives.

Stress's effects on hormone balance

The hypothalamic-pituitary-adrenal (HPA), sympathetic-adrenal-medullary (SAM), and hypothalamic-pituitary-gonadal (HPG) axes are three bodily systems that are impacted by stress that can significantly alter hormonal balance. Here's how hormonal balance may be impacted by stress:

1.Activation of the HPA Axis: The HPA axis is involved in a series of hormonal reactions that the body experiences in response to stress, both psychological and physical. Adrenocorticotropic hormone (ACTH) is released by the pituitary gland in response to stimulation by corticotropin-

releasing hormone (CRH) released by the
hypothalamus. The main stress hormone,
cortisol, is then produced by the adrenal
glands in response to an ACTH signal. High
cortisol levels promote energy availability,
reduce inflammation, and alter
immunological responses to help the body
deal with stress. On the other hand,
prolonged stress can cause the HPA axis to
become dysregulated, which can lead to
consistently elevated cortisol levels. This can
upset the hormonal balance and be a factor
in a number of health problems.

2. Effect on Gonadal Hormones: The HPG
axis, which controls the synthesis of sex
hormones like estrogen, progesterone, and
testosterone, can also be impacted by long-
term stress. Chronically high cortisol levels
can disrupt the hypothalamus's ability to
produce and release gonadotropin-releasing
hormone (GnRH), which in turn influences
the pituitary gland's ability to secrete

luteinizing hormone (LH) and follicle-stimulating hormone (FSH). Anovulation, irregular menstruation, problems with fertility in women, and changes in testosterone levels in both men and women can result from disruptions in the HPG axis.

3. Effects on Reproductive Function: Prolonged stress can change the way sex hormones are produced, secreted, and behave, which can interfere with regular reproductive processes. Hormonal imbalances brought on by stress can cause luteal phase abnormalities, irregular menstrual cycles, anovulation, and other menstrual diseases in women. Infertility, endometriosis, and polycystic ovarian syndrome (PCOS) are among the disorders that stress may exacerbate. Prolonged stress in men can have an impact on sperm quality and production, which lowers fertility.

4. Effects on Metabolism: Excessive cortisol levels brought on by long-term stress can also affect insulin sensitivity and metabolism, which can lead to metabolic disorders like insulin resistance, dyslipidemia, and abdominal obesity. These alterations in metabolism have the potential to worsen hormonal imbalances and raise the risk of developing diseases like metabolic syndrome, type 2 diabetes, and cardiovascular disease.

5. Effect on Mood and Behavior: Chronic stress-related hormonal imbalances can have an impact on mood, behavior, and cognitive performance. A high cortisol level may be a factor in anxiety, depression, irritability, and difficulty concentrating symptoms. In addition to impairing sleep quality, chronic stress can exacerbate hormone imbalance and worsen other health issues.

Chapter six

Medications to control symptoms

1.Birth control pills, or oral contraceptives:

• **Goal:** PCOS symptoms like irregular periods, acne, and hirsutism are commonly treated with oral contraceptives in order to normalize menstrual cycles.

• **Mode of Action:** Synthetic progestin and estrogen hormones, which restrict ovulation, control menstrual cycles, and lower testosterone levels, are present in combined oral contraceptives.

• **Advantages:** For women with PCOS, oral contraceptives can help control menstrual cycles, lower testosterone levels, treat acne, and lessen hirsutism. They also offer reliable birth control.

• **Examples:** There are other combinations of oral contraceptives on the market, including ethinyl estradiol with

norethindrone, drospirenone, or
levonorgestrel.

2. Anti-Androgen Supplements:

• **Goal:** Women with PCOS who experience signs of androgen excess, such as hirsutism and acne, can benefit from anti-androgen medicines.

• **Mechanism of Action:** By preventing androgens, or male hormones, from acting on specific tissues, anti-androgens lessen the symptoms associated with androgen excess.

• **Advantages:** For women with PCOS, anti-androgen drugs can assist with male-pattern hair loss, hirsutism, and acne.

• **As examples**, anti-androgen drugs such as spirolactone and cyproterone acetate are frequently prescribed to women with PCOS to treat hirsutism and acne.

3. Metformin:

• **Goal:** Women with PCOS who use metformin, an insulin-sensitizing drug, report improved insulin resistance and regular menstrual cycles.

• **Mechanism of Action:** Metformin improves insulin sensitivity in target tissues, increases peripheral glucose absorption, and reduces hepatic glucose synthesis.

• **Advantages:** For women with PCOS, metformin can help lower insulin levels, enhance glucose tolerance, control menstrual periods, and trigger ovulation. Additionally, it might lower testosterone levels and enhance the success of conception.

• As an illustration, metformin comes in formulations with both immediate and prolonged release.

4. Medication for Inducing Ovulation:

• **Goal:** For PCOS women attempting to conceive, ovulation induction drugs are utilized to induce ovulation.

• **Mechanism of Action:** By stimulating the ovaries to make and release eggs, ovulation induction medicines increase the likelihood of pregnancy.

- **Benefits:** Women with PCOS may benefit from ovulation induction drugs, which can help them ovulate and have better reproductive results. They can be used with other medications like metformin or assisted reproductive technologies (ART) or they can be used alone.

- **Examples:** Women with PCOS are frequently prescribed ovulation induction drugs, such as letrozole (Femara) and clomiphene citrate (Clomid).

5.Injections of gonadotropin:

- **Goal:** For PCOS women who have not responded to previous forms of treatment, gonadotropin injections provide an additional means of inducing ovulation.

- **Mode of Action:** Follicle-stimulating hormone (FSH) and/or luteinizing hormone (LH) found in gonadotropin injections encourage the ovaries to create and release eggs.

- **Benefits:** Injecting gonadotropin can help

women with PCOS trigger ovulation and enhance the success of their reproductive efforts. They are usually administered under the guidance of a fertility doctor and may increase the risk of ovarian hyperstimulation syndrome (OHSS) and multiple pregnancies.

• **Examples:** Drugs like recombinant FSH (rFSH) and human menopausal gonadotropin (hMG) are used in gonadotropin injections.

6. Additional Drugs:

• **Other medication** may be prescribed to treat particular PCOS symptoms or issues. Examples include acne treatments (topical retinoids, oral antibiotics), hair removal techniques (e.g., electrolysis, laser hair removal), and drugs to treat other co-occurring conditions (e.g., insulin-sensitizing agents for metabolic syndrome or type 2 diabetes).

.

hormonal birth control

Medications called hormonal contraceptives, sometimes referred to as birth control tablets, work by modifying the body's hormone levels to prevent conception. They contain synthetic forms of the hormones progestin and/or estrogen, which suppress ovulation, thicken cervical mucus to impede sperm penetration, and thin the lining of the uterus to stop a fertilized egg from implanting. Hormonal contraceptives are prescribed for a number of additional reasons besides their contraceptive effects, such as the treatment of acne, irregular menstruation, and symptoms of disorders like PCOS (Polycystic Ovary Syndrome). The many kinds of hormonal contraceptives are as follows:

1.Oral contraceptives combined (COCs):

• The hormones progestin and estrogen are both synthetically produced in COCs.

• During the course of a menstrual cycle, they are taken orally, usually once daily, for 21 to 28 days.

• Because COCs are available in a variety of formulations with varying progestin and estrogen dosages, customized treatment is possible.

• Tablets that combine progestins like levonorgestrel, norethindrone, desogestrel, drospirenone, or others with ethinyl estradiol are among the examples.

2. POPs, or progestin-only pills:

POPs, or mini-pills, are made up exclusively of progestin hormones.

• They are taken orally, without a break between pills, usually once a day.

• Women who are unable to utilize estrogen-containing contraceptives because of adverse effects or contraindications are frequently administered POPs.

• Tablets containing norgestrel, desogestrel, or norethindrone are among the examples.

3. Patch for contraception:

• The transdermal contraceptive patch is a method of delivering progestin and estrogen hormones through the skin.

• For three weeks, it is applied topically once a week to the skin. After that, a week without patches is allowed to allow for withdrawal bleeding.

• For women who prefer or cannot bear taking daily pills, the patch offers an oral alternative with comparable contraceptive efficacy and benefits to COCs.

4. Vaginal Contraceptive Ring:

• The flexible, transparent vaginal ring used for contraception is put into the vagina.

• It provides three weeks of contraception per ring by locally releasing the hormones progestin and estrogen.

• The user inserts the ring and takes it out

after three weeks. Thereafter, there is a one-week ring-free period to allow for withdrawal bleeding.

5. Intraperitoneal Contraceptives:

• Every three months, injectable contraceptives, such as Depo-Provera (medroxyprogesterone acetate), are given intramuscularly or subcutaneously.

• They offer highly effective long-acting contraception that just contains progestin hormones.

6. Contraceptives implanted:

• Small, flexible rods called implantable contraceptives, such Nexplanon (etonogestrel implant), are implanted beneath the skin of the upper arm.

• They continually produce progestin hormones for a number of years, which is a very effective kind of birth control.

When taken properly and regularly, hormonal contraceptives are quite successful at preventing pregnancy. They do not, however, offer protection against sexually transmitted diseases (STIs), hence condoms and other preventative measures are advised. Hormonal contraceptives are accessible with a prescription; a healthcare professional should prescribe and oversee the use of these medications based on each patient's unique needs, preferences, and medical history.

Anti-androgen drugs

A class of pharmaceuticals known as anti-androgens is intended to counteract the effects of androgens, or male sex hormones that are found in both men and women. Anti-androgen drugs are frequently recommended to treat symptoms of androgen excess, such as hirsutism (excessive hair growth), acne, and male-pattern hair loss, in the setting of diseases like PCOS (Polycystic Ovary Syndrome). These drugs function by either decreasing the production of androgens or inhibiting their activity. Here are a few anti-androgen drugs that are frequently prescribed:

1.spirolactone:

• Spironolactone is a diuretic that spares potassium while simultaneously having anti-androgenic qualities.

• It functions by preventing androgens from acting on cells, specifically at the androgen receptor sites in skin and hair follicles.

• Women with PCOS who experience hirsutism, acne, and female-pattern hair loss are frequently treated with spirolactone.

• Depending on the person's response and tolerance, the dosage may change and it is often given orally once or twice daily.

• Menstrual abnormalities, breast soreness, dizziness, and electrolyte imbalances are possible side effects.

2. Acetate of Cyproterone:

• A synthetic progestin with strong anti-androgenic qualities is cyproterone acetate.

• It functions by preventing androgens from acting on androgen receptor sites and by preventing the ovaries and adrenal glands from producing androgens.

• For PCOS-afflicted women, cyproterone acetate is frequently combined with estrogen in oral contraceptive pills to address symptoms of androgen excess, including acne and hirsutism.

• It can also be used in conjunction with other drugs or on its alone to treat androgenetic alopecia, or female pattern hair loss, in cases of severe hirsutism.

• Mood swings, liver function problems, breast discomfort, and irregular menstruation are possible side effects.

3. Flutamide:

• A nonsteroidal anti-androgen drug that competitively inhibits androgen receptors is called flutamide.

• It is mainly used to treat advanced prostate cancer in males, but it can also be used off-label to treat acne and hirsutism in PCOS-affected women.

• Flutamide is often given orally in divided dosages, frequently in conjunction with other hormonal drugs or an oral contraceptive pill.

• Reversible infertility, gastrointestinal problems, breast tenderness, and liver damage are possible side effects.

4. Finasteride:

• The 5-alpha reductase inhibitor drug finasteride prevents testosterone from being converted to dihydrotestosterone (DHT), which is a more potent form.

• It is mostly used to treat male-pattern hair loss and benign prostatic hyperplasia (BPH) in men; off-label use may also be utilized to treat hirsutism and female-pattern hair loss in PCOS-affected women.

Typically, finasteride is taken orally once day.

Chapter eight

Treatments for fertility for those trying to get pregnant

Fertility treatments may be required for PCOS (Polycystic Ovary Syndrome) patients who want to become pregnant in order to overcome ovulatory dysfunction and increase the likelihood of conception. The goals of these therapies are to maximize reproductive results, control menstrual cycles, and trigger ovulation. The following are a few typical fertility therapies for PCOS management:

1.Medication for Inducing Ovulation:

• The first-line treatment for anovulatory infertility in women with PCOS is ovulation induction medication.

• Two popular drugs used to induce ovulation are letrozole (Femara) and clomiphene citrate (Clomid).

• Follicle-stimulating hormone (FSH), luteinizing hormone (LH), and gonadotropin-releasing hormone (GnRH) are secreted more when clomiphene citrate blocks estrogen receptors in the hypothalamus. The ovaries are stimulated to generate and release eggs as a result.

• The aromatase inhibitor levozole inhibits the synthesis of estrogen, which increases the secretion of FSH and promotes the growth of follicles.

• Oral ovulation induction drugs are often used for five days at the onset of the menstrual cycle. The dosage is usually started low and increased dependent on the patient's reaction.

• During treatment cycles, ovarian response may be monitored using ultrasound and blood tests to evaluate follicular development and modify medication dosages as needed.

2. Injections of gonadotropin:

• Follicle-stimulating hormone (FSH) and/or luteinizing hormone (LH) are found in gonadotropin injections, which are used to directly activate the ovaries.

• Gonadotropin injections are usually administered in cases of severe anovulation or when oral medicines, such as letrozole or clomiphene citrate, have failed to induce ovulation.

• At the start of the menstrual cycle, they are given as subcutaneous injections every day for a few days. The dosages are modified based on the ovarian response, which is tracked by blood tests and ultrasounds.

• Compared to oral drugs, gonadotropin injections are associated with an increased risk of multiple pregnancies and ovarian hyperstimulation syndrome (OHSS).

3.IUI, or intrauterine insemination:

• To improve the likelihood of fertilization, prepared sperm are inserted directly into the uterus during ovulation by intrauterine insemination.

IUI and ovulation induction drugs can be used in tandem to maximize timing and boost the quantity of eggs that are accessible.

• IUI is a somewhat easy and non-invasive technique that is usually carried out in a medical professional's office.

• In cases of infertility that cannot be explained or when other reproductive therapies have failed, IUI may be advised.

4.IVF, or in vitro fertilization:

• One more sophisticated form of in vitro fertilization includes extracting numerous eggs from the ovaries, fertilizing them with sperm in a lab, and putting the resulting embryos into the uterus. This process is done by stimulating the ovaries with drugs to create many eggs.

• If a PCOS patient has not responded to previous fertility treatments, has additional fertility issues besides ovulatory dysfunction, or meets certain criteria for IVF, then IVF may be advised.

• Compared to IUI and ovulation induction

drugs, in vitro fertilization (IVF) is a more intrusive and costly treatment option, but it may have greater success rates, particularly in situations of severe infertility.

5.Changes in Lifestyle:

• Lifestyle changes, such as eating a balanced diet, exercising frequently, managing stress, abstaining from tobacco and excessive alcohol consumption, and keeping a healthy weight, can also enhance reproductive outcomes in PCOS patients in addition to medication therapies.

PCOS patients should receive customized fertility treatments that are tailored to their unique needs, preferences, and medical background. These treatments should be administered by a medical professional with experience managing PCOS and infertility. Throughout the course of treatment, close observation and assistance are necessary to maximize results and reduce hazards.

Medication to induce ovulation

For those suffering from ovulatory dysfunction and infertility due to PCOS (Polycystic Ovary Syndrome), ovulation induction drugs are a popular form of treatment. By encouraging the ovaries to create and release eggs, these drugs improve the likelihood of becoming pregnant. The following list of frequently prescribed ovulation induction drugs is used to treat PCOS:

1.Citrate clomiphene (Clomid):

• The ovulation-inducing agent clomiphene citrate is a selective estrogen receptor modulator (SERM).

• It functions by obstructing the hypothalamus's estrogen receptors, which increases the release of luteinizing hormone (LH), follicle-stimulating hormone (FSH), and gonadotropin-releasing hormone (GnRH).

• This promotes ovarian follicle growth and

maturation, which eventually results in ovulation.

• At the onset of the menstrual cycle, clomiphene citrate is normally taken orally for five days. The dosage is usually started low (e.g., 50 mg/day) and increased as necessary based on the individual's reaction.

• During treatment cycles, ovarian response may be monitored using ultrasound and blood tests to evaluate follicular development and modify medication dosages as needed.

• Mood swings, breast discomfort, ovarian enlargement, and hot flashes are common adverse effects of clomiphene citrate.

2. Letrozole: Also known as Femara

• An aromatase inhibitor drug called metronidazole is also prescribed off-label to PCOS-afflicted women in order to induce ovulation.

• The way it functions is by blocking the enzyme aromatase, which changes androgens like testosterone into estrogens like estradiol.

• Follicle development and secretion of follicle-stimulating hormone (FSH) are enhanced by letrozole due to its suppression of estrogen production.

Like clomiphene citrate, metronidazole is usually taken orally for five days at the start of the menstrual cycle.

• In women who do not respond to or tolerate clomiphene citrate, it may be used as an alternative for inducing ovulation.

• Headache, nausea, exhaustion, and hot flashes are possible side effects of letrozole.

3. Injections of gonadotropin:

• Follicle-stimulating hormone (FSH) and/or luteinizing hormone (LH) are found in gonadotropin injections, which are used to stimulate the ovaries directly.

• They are usually used in cases of severe anovulation or when oral medications like letrozole or clomiphene citrate have failed to induce ovulation.

• At the start of the menstrual cycle, injections of gonadotropin are given subcutaneously once a day for a few days.

• During treatment cycles, ovarian response is tracked with blood tests and ultrasounds, and dosages are modified accordingly.

• Compared to oral drugs, gonadotropin injections are associated with an increased risk of multiple pregnancies and ovarian hyperstimulation syndrome (OHSS).

Risks and adverse effects of possible medical interventions

People should be aware of the risks and possible side effects of any medical interventions for PCOS, including prescription drugs and infertility therapies. It's crucial to go over these with a medical professional before beginning treatment. The following are some possible risks and side effects of common PCOS medical interventions:

1.Ovulation Induction Medications (Clomiphene Citrate, Letrozole):

• Hot Flashes: Some individuals may experience hot flashes as a side effect of ovulation induction medications, particularly clomiphene citrate.

• Mood Swings: Changes in mood, including irritability and emotional sensitivity, may occur as a result of hormonal fluctuations induced by these medications.

• Ovarian Hyperstimulation Syndrome (OHSS): In rare cases, ovulation induction medications can lead to OHSS, a potentially serious condition characterized by enlarged ovaries, fluid accumulation in the abdomen, and electrolyte imbalances. Signs may be abdominal pain, vomiting, bloating, nausea, and difficult in breathing. Severe cases of OHSS may necessitate hospitalization and medical intervention.

2. Anti-androgen Medications (Spironolactone, Cyproterone Acetate):

• Menstrual Irregularities: Anti-androgen drugs may induce abnormalities in menstrual patterns, including breakthrough bleeding or amenorrhea (lack of menstruation).

• Breast soreness: Some persons may suffer breast soreness as a side effect of anti-androgen medicines.

• Electrolyte Imbalances: Spironolactone, in particular, is a potassium-sparing diuretic and may lead to electrolyte imbalances, especially if taken at high doses or in combination with other medications that affect potassium levels.

3. Fertility Treatments (Gonadotropin Injections, Intrauterine Insemination, In Vitro Fertilization):

• Multiple Pregnancies: Fertility treatments, especially those involving ovulation induction with gonadotropin injections, increase the risk of multiple pregnancies, including twins, triplets, or higher-order multiples.

• Ovarian Hyperstimulation Syndrome (OHSS): As mentioned earlier, fertility treatments involving ovarian stimulation with gonadotropin injections can lead to OHSS, a potentially serious condition that requires medical attention.

• Ectopic Pregnancy: Fertility treatments, particularly those involving assisted reproductive technologies such as in vitro fertilization (IVF), may slightly increase the risk of ectopic pregnancy, where the fertilized egg implants outside the uterus, usually in the fallopian tube.

• Emotional and Psychological Stress: Undergoing fertility treatments can be emotionally and psychologically challenging, leading to stress, anxiety, and depression in some individuals.

4. Other Medications and Interventions:

• Birth Control Pills: Hormonal contraceptives, including birth control pills, may have side effects such as nausea, headache, breast tenderness, and mood changes. They may also increase the risk of blood clots, particularly in individuals with certain risk factors.

• Metformin: Metformin, commonly used to improve insulin sensitivity in PCOS, may cause gastrointestinal side effects such as diarrhea, nausea, and abdominal discomfort, particularly when starting treatment or with higher doses.

• Surgical Interventions: In some cases, surgical interventions such as ovarian drilling or bariatric surgery may be recommended for individuals with PCOS. Risks associated with these procedures include bleeding, infection, and anesthesia-related complications. When thinking about medical treatments for PCOS, it's critical for patients to balance the advantages and disadvantages and share any worries with their physician. It is crucial to conduct frequent follow-up appointments and closely monitor any side effects that may occur during treatment. Furthermore, lifestyle changes like eating a balanced diet, staying physically active, and maintaining a healthy weight can enhance medical interventions and enhance the general health of PCOS patients.

Chapter nine

List of popular supplements for PCOS

People with PCOS (Polycystic Ovary Syndrome) frequently use a number of vitamins to assist control their symptoms and enhance their general health. While research on the usefulness of these supplements for PCOS is ongoing, some data suggests that they may have favorable effects in select situations. It's vital to contact with a healthcare provider before starting any new supplement program, as they can interfere with drugs or exacerbate certain health conditions. Here are some regularly used medicines for PCOS:

1.Inositol:

• Inositol is a form of sugar alcohol that is found in numerous foods and also created by the body.

• Studies suggest that inositol supplementation may enhance insulin sensitivity, regulate menstrual cycles, and lessen symptoms of hirsutism and acne in women with PCOS.

• Two types of inositol often used for PCOS are myo-inositol and D-chiro-inositol, often taken together in a specified ratio.

2. Vitamin D:

• Vitamin D insufficiency is common in persons with PCOS and may be connected with insulin resistance, inflammation, and other metabolic abnormalities.

• Supplementing with vitamin D may help improve insulin sensitivity, regulate menstrual cycles, and reduce inflammation in certain persons with PCOS.

• Optimal vitamin D levels should be maintained through a mix of sunshine exposure, food sources, and supplementation if necessary.

3. Omega-3 Fatty Acids:

• Omega-3 fatty acids, found in fatty fish (e.g., salmon, mackerel), flaxseeds, and walnuts, have anti-inflammatory qualities and may help lower inflammation associated with PCOS.

• Supplementing with omega-3 fatty acids may help improve lipid profiles, reduce insulin resistance, and alleviate symptoms of depression and anxiety in individuals with PCOS.

4. N-Acetyl Cysteine (NAC):

• N-acetyl cysteine is a precursor to glutathione, a strong antioxidant that helps protect cells from oxidative damage.

• Studies suggest that NAC administration may enhance insulin sensitivity, lower androgen levels, and improve ovulation and menstrual regularity in women with PCOS.

5. Chromium:

• The trace mineral chromium is involved in insulin sensitivity and glucose metabolism.

• According to certain research, chromium supplements may help PCOS patients become more insulin sensitive and less insulin resistant.

• Chromium picolinate is a regularly utilized type of chromium supplementation.

6. The mineral magnesium

• The body uses magnesium as a necessary mineral for several metabolic processes, such as insulin signaling and glucose metabolism.

• There is some evidence that supplementing with magnesium may help PCOS patients become less insulin resistant and more sensitive to insulin.

• The two most popular types of magnesium supplementation are magnesium citrate and magnesium glycinate.

7. Berberine:

• A number of plants, including Oregon grape, goldenseal, and barberry, contain the chemical berberine.

• Research indicates that supplementing with berberine may help women with PCOS control their menstrual cycles, lower their levels of testosterone, and increase their sensitivity to insulin.

8. Folate, or acid folic

• Folate, sometimes referred to as vitamin B9, is necessary for cell division and DNA synthesis.

• Some evidence suggests that folate supplementation may assist enhance ovarian function and reproductive outcomes in people with PCOS.

• The synthetic form of folate that is frequently seen in supplements is called folic acid.

9. Vitamin B12:

• DNA synthesis it helps form the red blood cell, and neuron function all depend on vitamin B12.

• A vitamin B12 deficiency may be present in some PCOS patients, which may exacerbate symptoms including exhaustion and neuropathy.

• Giving PCOS sufferers a vitamin B12 supplement may help reduce these symptoms and improve their general health.

10. Probiotics:

• Probiotics are good bacteria that support the preservation of a balanced population of gut microflora.

• According to some research, probiotic supplements may benefit PCOS sufferers' gut health, lower inflammation, and lessen the symptoms of metabolic syndrome.

The use of acupuncture

Thin needles are inserted into particular body locations during acupuncture, a kind of traditional Chinese medicine (TCM), to stimulate Qi (pronounced "chee"), the body's energy flow, and aid in healing. Although acupuncture has been used for hundreds of years to treat a wide range of illnesses, research is currently being done to see whether it may effectively treat PCOS (polycystic ovarian syndrome). What is known about acupuncture in relation to PCOS is as follows:

1. Menstrual Cycle Regulation: Research indicates that acupuncture may assist in regulating menstrual periods and encouraging ovulation in PCOS-affected women. Acupuncture may affect hormone levels, enhance blood flow to the ovaries, and bring the reproductive system back into balance by stimulating particular acupuncture points.

2. Enhancement of Hormonal Balance: Because acupuncture can affect the levels of insulin, estrogen, progesterone, and androgens (such as testosterone), it has been suggested as a supplemental treatment for PCOS. Acupuncture may help relieve problems including irregular periods, hirsutism (excessive hair growth), and acne by focusing on particular acupuncture sites linked to hormone balance.

3. Reduction of Insulin Resistance: One

metabolic characteristic of PCOS that is frequently present is insulin resistance, which contributes to symptoms like weight gain, difficulties reducing weight, and an elevated risk of type 2 diabetes. According to some study, acupuncture may influence insulin signaling pathways and glucose metabolism, which could assist people with PCOS experience improvements in insulin sensitivity and decreases in insulin resistance.

4. Handling Stress and Anxiety: People with PCOS frequently experience stress, anxiety, and sadness that is associated with their disease. This can have a substantial influence on mental health. Research has demonstrated that acupuncture can induce the release of endorphins and other neurotransmitters, which can have a relaxing and stress-relieving impact. Acupuncture may help enhance general wellbeing in PCOS patients by encouraging relaxation and lowering stress levels.

5. Enhancement of Fertility: For women with PCOS undergoing assisted reproductive technologies (ART) like in vitro fertilization (IVF) or intrauterine insemination (IUI), acupuncture is frequently utilized as a supplemental therapy. Enhancing blood flow to the uterus, controlling hormone levels, and lowering stress levels during fertility treatments are all possible benefits of acupuncture that may increase the likelihood of conception and a healthy pregnancy. Although some studies point to possible advantages of acupuncture for PCOS, additional investigation is required to completely comprehend its efficacy and mechanisms of action. People who are thinking about trying acupuncture for PCOS should definitely speak with a registered and skilled acupuncturist and collaborate with their doctor to incorporate acupuncture into their entire treatment plan. As long as sterile needles and the proper techniques are used by qualified practitioners, acupuncture is usually regarded as safe. But not everyone will benefit from it, and each person's reaction to acupuncture is unique.

Coping mechanisms for anxiety, depression, and problems with body image

The following coping mechanisms could be useful in handling these emotional difficulties:

1. Seek expert Assistance: It's critical to get treatment from a mental health expert, such as a therapist or counselor, if you're experiencing anxiety, sadness, or problems with your body image. In order to examine your ideas and feelings, acquire coping mechanisms, and create symptom management plans, therapy can offer a secure and accepting environment.

2. Engage in Mindfulness and Meditation: These techniques can help lower anxiety, ease the symptoms of depression, and encourage acceptance of one's body. Allocate a specific period of time on a daily basis for mindfulness practices, such guided meditation, body scans, or deep breathing. Concentrate on staying in the present and objectively examining your thoughts and feelings.

3. Exercise Frequently: Research has indicated that regular physical activity improves mental and emotional well-being. Include exercise on a regular basis in your schedule and find things that you enjoy doing. Moving your body can help lower anxiety, elevate mood, and enhance body image, whether you do it through yoga, dancing, walking, or swimming.

4. Exercise Self-Compassion: Show yourself kindness and compassion, particularly when you're having trouble with unfavorable feelings and thoughts. Engage in self-care routines that support your body, mind, and soul.

5. Identify and combat negative ideas and perceptions you may have about your appearance and yourself. Utilize cognitive behavioral strategies to develop more realistic and balanced viewpoints and to reframe negative thought patterns. Concentrate on your advantages, successes, and admirable traits.

Chapter ten

Recognizing the connections between PCOS and other medical disorders

PCOS (polycystic ovarian syndrome) has direct and indirect associations with a number of different medical disorders. Comprehending these correlations is crucial for all-encompassing supervision and tackling possible health hazards. The following are a few typical medical issues linked to PCOS:

1. Diabetes and Insulin Resistance: One of the main characteristics of PCOS is insulin resistance, which results in high blood sugar levels because the body's cells become less sensitive to insulin. This can develop into type 2 diabetes and prediabetes over time. Diabetes is more likely to strike people with PCOS, particularly if they are obese or overweight. Preventing diabetes and its complications requires managing insulin resistance with medication, dietary changes, and routine monitoring.

2. Metabolic syndrome raise the risk of heart disease, stroke, and type 2 diabetes. Typical symptoms include abnormal cholesterol levels, elevated blood sugar, high blood pressure, and central obesity. Metabolic syndrome is thought to be predisposed by PCOS, especially in women who have abdominal obesity and insulin resistance. For PCOS patients, weight control, a good diet, and physical exercise are key lifestyle therapies that lower their chance of developing metabolic syndrome.

3. Cardiovascular Disease: Heart attacks, strokes, and coronary artery disease (CVD) are among the conditions for which PCOS increases the risk. This increased risk is caused by a number of factors, including insulin resistance, obesity, dyslipidemia (abnormal lipid levels), and hypertension. A heart-healthy diet, quitting smoking, managing other risk factors, and regular exercise are all crucial lifestyle changes that help lower the risk of CVD in those with PCOS.

4. Endometrial hyperplasia and Cancer: PCOS is linked to anovulation, irregular menstrual periods, and unopposed estrogen exposure. These factors can cause the uterine lining to thicken, a condition known as endometrial hyperplasia, which raises the risk of endometrial cancer. A higher risk may apply to women with PCOS who have irregular or nonexistent menstrual cycles. Hormonal treatments, including progestin therapy or combined oral contraceptives, can help control menstrual periods and lower the risk of cancer and endometrial hyperplasia.

5. Obstructive Sleep Apnea (OSA): A sleep condition marked by recurrent bouts of total or partial upper airway obstruction during sleep, OSA is more common in those with PCOS. Obesity, insulin resistance, and hormonal imbalances are among the factors that lead to the development of OSA in PCOS patients. To improve sleep quality and lower cardiovascular risk in PCOS patients, screening for OSA and treating risk factors with weight management, positional therapy, continuous positive airway pressure (CPAP), or other treatments is crucial.

6. Mood Disorders: An elevated risk of mood disorders, such as eating disorders, anxiety, and depression, is linked to PCOS. Mood disorders may be exacerbated by the hormonal and metabolic imbalances linked to PCOS as well as the psychosocial effects of the illness. An integral part of managing PCOS is conducting mood disorder screenings and offering appropriate psychological therapies and support, including support groups, CBT, and counseling.

7. Reproductive Health Complications: PCOS can affect a woman's ability to conceive and maintain a healthy pregnancy, which can result in problems like infertility, miscarriage, and pregnancy complications like gestational diabetes and preeclampsia. Preconception counseling, health optimization, and close collaboration with healthcare experts are recommended for women with PCOS who intend to become pregnant in order to control their disease and lower the likelihood of pregnancy difficulties.

Regular health check and preventive care are essential.

For those with PCOS (polycystic ovary syndrome), routine health monitoring and preventative care are essential to managing the illness well, avoiding complications, and enhancing general wellbeing. For those with PCOS, routine health monitoring and preventative care are crucial for the following reasons:

1.Early Detection and Diagnosis: PCOS and

related health issues can be identified and diagnosed early thanks to routine health monitoring

2. Handling Symptoms and Health Risks: Polycystic Ovary Syndrome (PCOS) is linked to a number of symptoms and health risks, including as diabetes, insulin resistance, heart disease, and issues with reproduction. Frequent health monitoring enables medical professionals to modify treatment plans and treatments as necessary to control symptoms and lower health risks by keeping track of changes in hormone levels, metabolic parameters, and symptoms.

3. Screening for Complications: Diabetes, heart disease, endometrial hyperplasia, and mood disorders are among the health issues that people with PCOS are more likely to experience. In order to identify these issues early and enable prompt intervention and therapy, routine health monitoring involves screening tests and evaluations.

4. Optimization of therapy and Management: Frequent health monitoring gives medical professionals important information for PCOS therapy and management plan optimization. Individualized treatment programs that are suited to each patient's needs and objectives are made possible by the monitoring of hormone levels, metabolic parameters, and other health indicators.

5. Preventive measures for health: Preventive treatment is essential for lowering the chance of problems from PCOS and enhancing long-term health. This could involve behavioral therapies (like stress reduction and quitting smoking), medication management (such insulin-sensitizing agents and hormonal contraceptives), and lifestyle changes (including maintaining a healthy diet, getting regular exercise, and managing weight).

6. Fertility Planning and Pregnancy

Management: To maximize fertility outcomes and guarantee a healthy pregnancy, people with PCOS who are planning a pregnancy or who are already pregnant must have frequent health monitoring. Monitoring reproductive health parameters, ovulation, menstrual periods, and hormone levels makes it possible to detect potential problems or complications early on and provide the right care and support.

7. Psychological Support and Counseling: Anxiety, depression, and problems with body image are just a few of the symptoms of PCOS can have a major influence on mental health. In order to address the emotional and psychosocial components of PCOS and support mental health, routine health monitoring offers opportunity for psychological assessment and help, such as counseling, therapy, and support groups.

Diabetes type 2

Hyperglycemia, or elevated blood sugar, is a hallmark of type 2 diabetes, a long-term metabolic condition brought on by insulin resistance and relative insulin insufficiency. The pancreas secretes the hormone insulin, which aids in the uptake of glucose into cells for use as fuel or storage. This helps control blood sugar levels. Elevated blood sugar levels occur when cells in type 2 diabetics grow resistant to the effects of insulin, and the pancreas may not generate enough insulin to overcome this resistance.

Here are some essential details regarding type 2 diabetes:

1.Risk Factors: A number of variables raise the possibility of type 2 diabetes, such as:

• A family background of diabetes

• Being overweight or obese, particularly

having too much belly fat

- A sedentary way of life
- Unhealthy diet heavy in sugar, saturated fats, and processed carbs
- Age (risk rises with advancing years, especially beyond 45)
- Ethnicity (certain ethnic groups are more vulnerable than others, including Asians, Native Americans, African Americans, and Hispanics).
- A history of prediabetes or gestational diabetes
- PCOS, or polycystic ovarian syndrome

2.Type 2 diabetes symptoms can appear gradually and include:

- Increased urination and thirst
- Tiredness
- Hazed vision
- Sluggish healing of wounds
- Recurrent infections, like skin or urinary tract infections
- Neuropathy causing tingling or numbness

in the hands or feet

3.Diagnosis: Blood tests measuring hemoglobin A1c (HbA1c) levels, the oral glucose tolerance test (OGTT), or fasting blood sugar levels are used to diagnose type 2 diabetes. If the HbA1c is 6.5% or more, the OGTT reveals blood sugar levels of 200 mg/dL or higher, or the fasting blood sugar is 126 mg/dL or higher, the diagnosis of diabetes is usually confirmed.

4.Complications: Uncontrolled type 2 diabetes can result in a number of issues, such as:

• Cardiovascular disorders (stroke, heart disease)

• Neuropathy (injury to nerves)

Nephropathy: injury to the kidneys

Retinopathy: injury to the eyes

• Foot issues (ulcers, diabetic neuropathy)

• Skin disorders (fungal and bacterial infections)

• Dental issues (tooth loss, gum disease)

- Dysfunctional relationships
- Impaired cognitive function

5.Management and Treatment: The goals of type 2 diabetes treatment are to better general health, avoid complications, and regulate blood sugar levels. It might consist of:

- Changes in lifestyle: a balanced diet, frequent exercise, and weight control
- Oral drugs: GLP-1 receptor agonists, DPP-4 inhibitors, SGLT2 inhibitors, sulfonylureas, and metformin
- Medication that can be injected: GLP-1 receptor agonists, insulin
- Blood sugar monitoring: Consistently checking blood sugar levels
- Routine check-ups: keeping an eye out for issues and modifying care as necessary
- Information and assistance: counseling, support groups, and instruction on diabetes self-management

6.Prevention: By making lifestyle changes

that lower the risk factors linked to the disease, type 2 diabetes can be substantially avoided. These include maintaining a healthy weight, exercising frequently, abstaining from tobacco use, limiting alcohol intake, and choosing a diet high in fruits, vegetables, whole grains, and lean proteins.